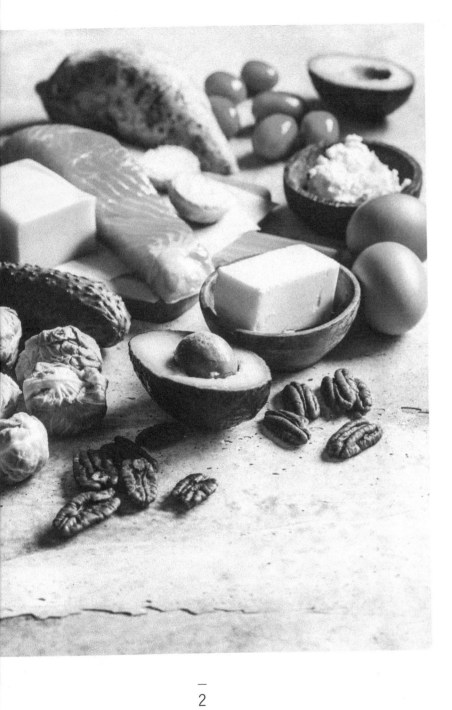

KETO

COOKBOOK

Low Carb Recipes for a Keto Diet an
Lifestyle

JILL FOX

Table of Contents

Sommario

5

Introduction

The ketogenic diet, or keto diet, is a low carb, high-fat diet that gives many health benefits.

Many studies show that this sort of diet can assist you to reduce and improve your health.

Ketogenic diets may even have benefits against diabetes, cancer, epilepsy, and Alzheimer's disease.

What is a ketogenic diet?

The ketogenic diet is low carb, a high-fat diet that shares many similarities with the Atkins and low carb diets.

It involves drastically reducing carbohydrate intake and replacing it with fat. This reduction in carbs puts your body into a metabolic state called ketosis.

When this happens, your body becomes incredibly efficient at burning fat for energy. It also turns fat into ketones within the liver, which may supply energy for the brain

Ketogenic diets can cause significant reductions in blood glucose and insulin levels. This, alongside the increased ketones, has some health benefits.

—
7

Different types of ketogenic diets

There are several versions of the ketogenic diet, including:

The standard ketogenic diet (SKD): This is often a low carb, moderate protein, and high-fat diet. It typically contains 70% fat, 20% protein, and only 10% carbs (9Trusted Source).

The cyclical ketogenic diet (CKD): This diet involves periods of upper carb refeeds, like 5 ketogenic days followed by 2 high carb days.

The targeted ketogenic diet (TKD): This diet allows you to feature carbs around workouts.

High protein ketogenic diet: this is often almost like a typical ketogenic diet, but includes more protein. The ratio is usually 60% fat, 35% protein, and 5% carbs.

However, only the quality and high protein ketogenic diets are studied extensively. Cyclical or targeted ketogenic diets are more advanced methods and are primarily employed by bodybuilders or athletes.

What is ketosis?

Ketosis may be a metabolic state during which your body uses fat for fuel rather than carbs.

It occurs once you significantly reduce your consumption of carbohydrates, limiting your body's supply of glucose (sugar), which is that the main source of energy for the cells.

Following a ketogenic diet is that the best thanks to entering ketosis. Generally, this involves limiting carb consumption to around 20 to 50 grams per day and filling abreast of fats, like meat, fish, eggs, nuts, and healthy oils

It's also important to moderate your protein consumption, this is often because protein can be converted into glucose if consumed in high amounts, which can slow your transition into ketosis

Practicing intermittent fasting could also assist you to enter ketosis faster. There are many various sorts of intermittent fasting, but the foremost common method involves limiting food intake to around 8 hours per day and fasting for the remaining 16 hours

Blood, urine, and breath tests are available, which may help determine whether you've entered ketosis by measuring the number of ketones produced by your body.

Certain symptoms can also indicate that you've entered ketosis, including increased thirst, dry mouth, frequent urination, and decreased hunger or appetite

Ketogenic diets can help you lose weight

A ketogenic diet is also an effective solution for losing weight and decreasing risk factors for disease.

Research has shown that the ketogenic diet can be very effective for weight loss as a low-fat diet.

What's more, the diet is so rich that you can lose weight without needing to count calories or track your food intake.

An analysis of 13 studies revealed that following a low-carb ketogenic diet was slightly superior for long-term weight loss compared to a low-fat diet.

It also led to a reduction in diastolic blood pressure and triglyceride levels.

Other health benefits of keto

- The ketogenic diet originated as a method of treating neurological diseases such as epilepsy.
- Studies have now shown that this diet may have benefits for a wide variety of different health conditions:

- Heart disease. The ketogenic diet can help improve risk factors such as body fat, HDL (good) cholesterol levels, blood pressure, and blood sugar.

- Cancer. Diet is currently being explored as an adjunct treatment for cancer because it may help slow tumor growth.

- Alzheimer's disease. The keto diet may help reduce the symptoms of Alzheimer's disease and slow its progression.

- Epilepsy. Research has shown that the ketogenic diet can cause significant reductions in seizures in epileptic children.

- Parkinson's disease. Although more research is needed, one study found that the diet helped improve symptoms of Parkinson's disease.

- Polycystic ovary syndrome. The ketogenic diet may help reduce insulin levels, which may play a key role in polycystic ovary syndrome.

- Brain injury. Some research suggests that the diet may improve the outcomes of traumatic brain injuries.

However, keep in mind that research in many of these areas is far from conclusive.

Foods to avoid

Any food high in carbohydrates should be reduced.

Here is a list of foods that should be reduced or eliminated on a ketogenic diet:

sugary foods: soda, juice, smoothies, cake, ice cream, candy, etc.

grains or starches: wheat products, rice, pasta, cereals, etc.

fruits: all fruits, except small portions of berries such as strawberries

beans or legumes: peas, beans, lentils, chickpeas, etc.

root and tuber vegetables: potatoes, sweet potatoes, carrots, parsnips, etc.

low-fat or diet products: low-fat mayonnaise, salad dressings, and condiments

some condiments or sauces: barbecue sauce, honey mustard, teriyaki sauce, ketchup, etc.

unhealthy fats: processed vegetable oils, mayonnaise, etc.

alcohol: beer, wine, liquor, mixed drinks

sugar-free diet foods: sugar-free candy, syrups, puddings, sweeteners, desserts, etc.

Foods to eat

You should focus most of your meals on these foods:

meat: red meat, steak, ham, sausage, bacon, chicken, and turkey

fatty fish: salmon, trout, tuna, and mackerel

eggs: whole pastured eggs or omega-3s

butter and cream: grass-fed butter and heavy cream

cheese: non-processed cheeses such as cheddar, goat, cream, blue, or mozzarella cheese

nuts and seeds: almonds, walnuts, flaxseeds, pumpkin seeds, chia seeds, etc.

healthy oils: extra virgin olive oil, coconut oil, and avocado oil

avocado: whole avocado or freshly made guacamole

low carb vegetables: green vegetables, tomatoes, onions, peppers, etc.

seasonings: salt, pepper, herbs, and spices

It's best to base your diet primarily on whole, single-ingredient foods. Here's a list of 44 healthy low-carb foods.

Healthy keto snacks

In case you get the urge to eat between meals, here are some healthy, keto-approved snacks:

fatty meat or fish

cheese

a handful of nuts or seeds

keto sushi bites

olives

one or two hard-boiled or deviled eggs

keto-friendly snack bars

90 percent dark chocolate

whole Greek yogurt mixed with nut butter and cocoa powder

peppers and guacamole

strawberries and plain cottage cheese

celery with salsa and guacamole

beef jerky

smaller portions of leftover meals

fat bombs

Keto tips and tricks

Although starting the ketogenic diet can be difficult, there are several tips and tricks you can use to make it easier.

Start by familiarizing yourself with food labels and checking the grams of fat, carbohydrates, and fiber to determine how your favorite foods can fit into your diet.

Planning your meals can also be beneficial and can help you save extra time during the week.

Tips for eating out on a ketogenic diet

Many restaurant meals can be made keto-friendly.

Most restaurants offer some type of meat or fish dish. Order this food and replace any high-carb food with extra vegetables.

Egg meals are also a good option, such as an omelet or eggs and bacon.

Another favorite meal is burgers without a bun. You could also replace the fries with veggies. Add extra avocado, cheese, bacon, or eggs.

In Mexican restaurants, you can enjoy any type of meat with extra cheese, guacamole, salsa, and sour cream.

For dessert, ask for a tray of mixed cheeses or berries with cream.

At least, in the beginning, it's crucial to eat until you're full and avoid cutting calories too much. Usually, a ketogenic diet involves weight loss without intentional calorie restriction.

In this Keto cookbook, you can organize your Keto diet with the different dishes you'll find for meals throughout the day. Enjoy!

Breakfast

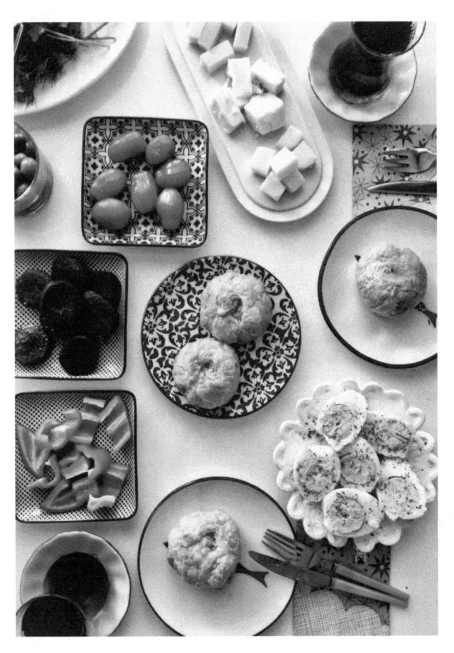

Cheesy Breakfast Muffins

Preparation Time: 15 minutes
Cooking Time: 12 minutes
Servings: 6

Ingredients:
4 tablespoons melted butter
3/4 tablespoon baking powder
cup almond flour
large eggs, lightly beaten
2 ounces cream cheese mixed with 2 tablespoons heavy whipping cream
A handful of shredded Mexican blend cheese

Directions:
Preheat the oven to 400°F. Grease 6 muffin tin cups with melted butter and set aside. Combine the baking powder and almond flour in a bowl. Stir well and set aside. Stir together four tablespoons melted butter, eggs, shredded cheese, and cream cheese in a separate bowl. The egg and the dry mixture must be combined using a hand mixer to beat until it is creamy and well blended. The mixture must be scooped into the greased muffin cups evenly.
Baking time: 12 minutes

Nutrition:
Calories: 214
Fat: 15.6g
Fiber: 3.1g
Carbohydrates: 5.1 g
Protein: 9.5 g

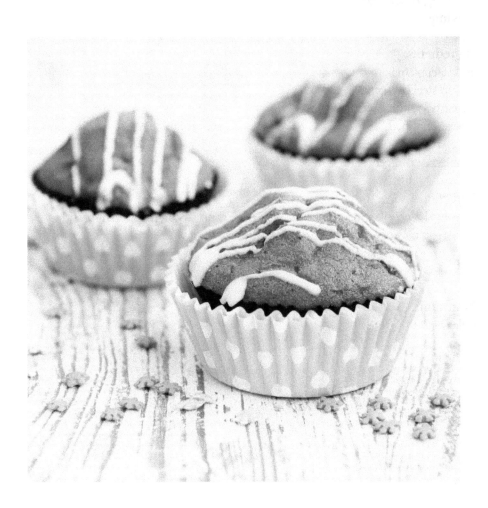

Pear and Maple Oatmeal

Preparation time: 10 minutes
Cooking time: 7 hours
Servings: 2

Ingredients:
and ½ cups milk
½ cup steel cut oats
½ teaspoon vanilla extract
1 pear, chopped
½ teaspoon maple extract
1 tablespoon sugar

Directions:
In your slow cooker, combine milk with oats, vanilla, pear, maple extract and sugar, stir, cover and cook on Low for 7 hours.
Divide into bowls and serve for breakfast.
Enjoy!

Nutrition:
Calories 200,
Fat 5,
Fiber 7,
Carbs 14, Protein 4

Sugary German Oatmeal

Preparation time: 10 minutes
Cooking time: 8 hours
Servings: 2

Ingredients:
Cooking spray
1 cup steel cut oats
3 cups water
6 ounces coconut milk
2 tablespoons cocoa powder
1 tablespoon brown sugar 1 tablespoon coconut, shredded

Directions:
Grease your slow cooker with cooking spray, add oats, water, milk, cocoa powder, sugar and shredded coconut, stir, cover and cook on Low for 8 hours. Stir oatmeal one more time, divide into 2 bowls and serve for breakfast. Enjoy!

Nutrition:
Calories 200,
Fat 4,
Fiber 5,
Carbs 17, Protein 5

Banana oatmeal

Preparation time: 5 minutes
Cooking time: 8 hours
Servings: 4

Ingredients:
Steel cut oats – 1 cup
Mashed ripe banana – 1
Chopped walnuts – ¼ cup
Skim milk – 2 cups
Water – 2 cups
Flax seed meal – 2 tablespoon
Cinnamon – 2 teaspoon
Vanilla – 1 teaspoon
Nutmeg – ½ teaspoon
Salt – ½ teaspoon
Banana slices – for garnish
Chopped walnuts – for garnish

Directions:-
Combine all the ingredients in a slow cooker except the banana slices and walnuts.
Cook covered for 8 hours on low.
Stir well.
Serve topped with walnuts and banana slices.

Nutrition:
290 Cal,
8 g total fat (7 g sat. fat),
2 mg cholesterol,
366 mg sodium, 42 g carb.
6.6g fiber,
11 g protein.

Romano Zucchini Cups

Preparation time: 10 minutes
Cooking time: 15 minutes
Servings: 4

Ingredients:
1 teaspoon sea salt
(½-pound / 227-g) zucchini, grated
½ cup almond flour
eggs, beaten
1 cup Romano cheese, grated

Directions:
Place the salt and grated zucchini in a bowl; let it sit for 15 minutes, squeeze using a cheesecloth and discard the liquid.

Now, stir in the almond flour, eggs, and Romano cheese. Spritz a 12cup mini-muffin pan with cooking spray.

Bake in the preheated oven for 15 minutes until the surface is no longer wet to the touch. Let them cool about 5 minutes to set up. Bon appétit!

Nutrition:
calories: 225 f
fat: 18.0g
protein: 13.4g
carbs: 3.0g
net carbs: 1.5g
fiber: 1.5g

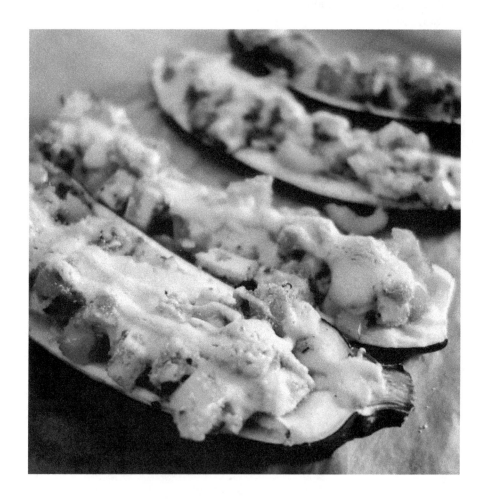

Spicy Cauliflower Steaks with Steamed Green Beans

Preparation Time: 15 minutes
Cooking Time: 20 minutes
Servings: 4

Ingredients:
2 heads cauliflower, sliced lengthwise into 'steaks.'
1/4 cup olive oil
1/4 cup chili sauce
2 tsp. erythritol
Salt and black pepper to taste
2 shallots, diced
bunch green beans, trimmed
tbsp. fresh lemon juice
1 cup of water Dried parsley to garnish

Directions:
In a bowl or container, mix the olive oil, chili sauce, and erythritol. Brush the cauliflower with the mixture. Grill for 6 minutes. Flip the cauliflower, cook further for 6 minutes. Let the water boil, place the green beans in a sieve, and set over the steam from the boiling water. Cover with a clean napkin to keep the steam trapped in the sieve. Cook for 6 minutes. After, remove to a bowl and toss with lemon juice. Remove the grilled caulis to a plate; sprinkle with salt, pepper, shallots, and parsley. Serve with the steamed green beans.

Nutrition:
Calories: 329
Fat: 10.4g
Fiber: 3.1g
Carbohydrates:4.2 g
Protein: 8.4g

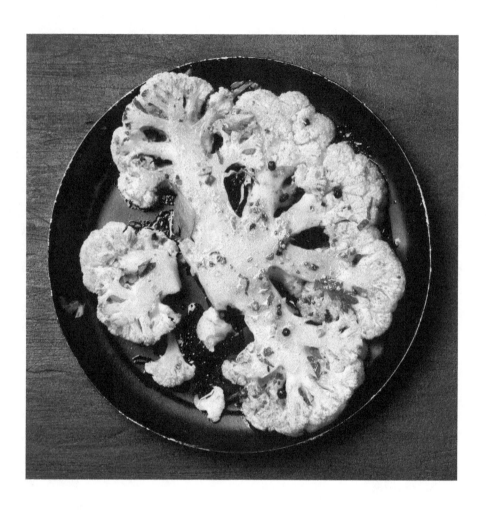

Chicken

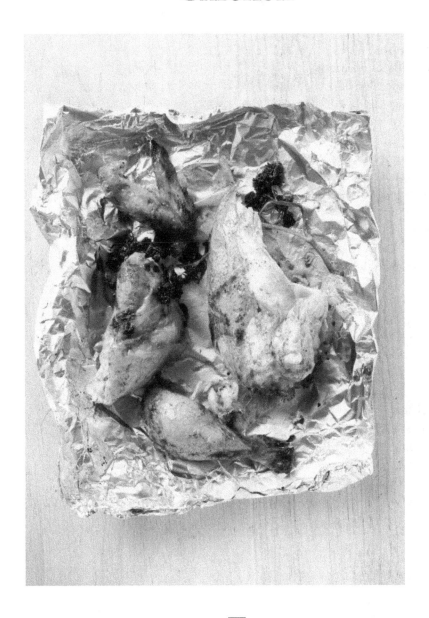

Chicken Spinach Salad

Preparation Time: 15 minutes
Cooking Time: 0 minutes
Servings: 3

Ingredients:
2 1/2 cups of spinach
4 1/2 ounces of boiled chicken
boiled eggs
1/2 cup of chopped cucumber
slices of bacon
1 small avocado
1 tablespoon olive oil
1/2 teaspoon of coconut oil
Pinch of Salt
Pepper

Directions:
Dice the boiled eggs.
Slice boiled chicken, bacon, avocado, spinach, cucumber, and combine them in a bowl. Then add diced boiled eggs.
Drizzle with some oil. Mix well.
Add salt and pepper to taste.
Enjoy.

Nutrition:
Calories: 265
Fat: 9.5g
Fiber: 10.5g
Carbohydrates:3.3 g
Protein: 14.1 g

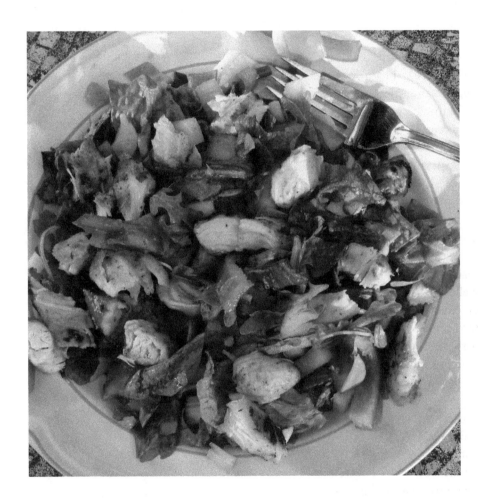

Baised Chicken in Italian Tomato Sauce

Preparation Time: 15 minutes
Cooking Time: 4 hrs.
Servings: 4

Ingredients:
1/4 cup olive oil, divided
4 (4-ounce / 113-g) boneless chicken thighs
Pepper and salt
1/2 cup chicken stock
4 ounces (113 g) julienned oil-packed sun-dried tomatoes
(28-ounce / 794-g) can sodium-free diced tomatoes
tablespoons dried oregano
2 tablespoons minced garlic
Red pepper flakes, to taste 2 tablespoons chopped fresh parsley

Directions:
Heat oil then put the chicken thighs in the skillet and sprinkle salt and black pepper to season. Sear the chicken thighs for 10 minutes or until well browned. Flip them halfway through the cooking time. Put the chicken thighs, stock, tomatoes, oregano, garlic, and red pepper flakes into the slow cooker. Stir to coat the chicken thighs well. High cook for 4 hrs. Transfer the chicken thighs to four plates. Pour the sauce which remains in the slow cooker over the chicken thighs and top with fresh parsley before serving warm.

Nutrition:
Calories: 464
Fat: 12.1g
Fiber: 8.5g
Carbohydrates:6.4 g
Protein: 13.1g

Italian Asiago and Pepper Stuffed Turkey

Preparation time: 15 minutes
Cooking time: 50 minutes
Servings: 62 tablespoons extra-virgin olive oil

Ingredients:
tablespoon Italian seasoning mix
Sea salt and freshly ground black pepper, to season
garlic cloves, sliced
6 ounces (170 g) Asiago cheese, sliced
2 bell peppers, thinly sliced
1½ pounds (680 g) turkey breasts
2 tablespoons Italian parsley, roughly chopped

Directions:
Brush the sides and bottom of a casserole dish with 1 tablespoon of extra-virgin olive oil. Preheat an oven to 360°F (182°C).
Sprinkle the turkey breast with the Italian seasoning mix, salt, and black pepper on all sides.
Make slits in each turkey breast and stuff with garlic, cheese, and bell peppers.
Drizzle the turkey breasts with the remaining tablespoon of olive oil.
Bake in the preheated oven for 50 minutes or until an instant-read thermometer registers 165°F (74°C).
Garnish with Italian parsley and serve warm. Bon appétit!

Nutrition:
calories: 350
fat: 22.3g
protein: 32.1g
carbs: 3.0g
net carbs: 2.4g
fiber: 0.6g

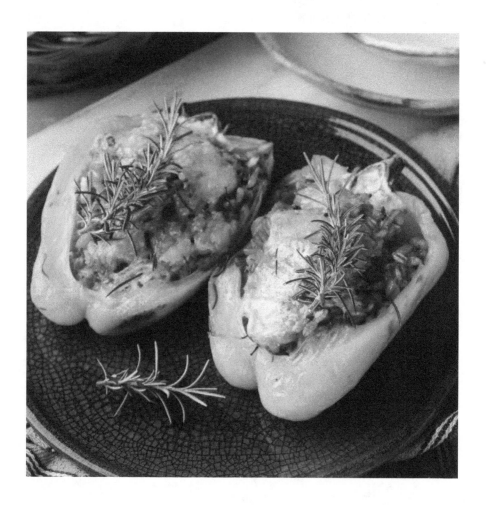

Herbed Balsamic Turkey

Preparation time: 15 minutes
Cooking time: 15 minutes
Servings: 2

Ingredients:
1 turkey drumstick, skinless and boneless
1 tablespoon balsamic vinegar
1 tablespoon whiskey
3 tablespoons olive oil
1 tablespoon stone ground mustard
½ teaspoon tarragon
1 teaspoon rosemary
1 teaspoon sage
1 garlic clove, pressed
Kosher salt and ground black pepper, to season
1 brown onion, peeled and chopped

Directions:
Place the turkey drumsticks in a ceramic dish. Toss them with the balsamic vinegar, whiskey, olive oil, mustard, tarragon, rosemary, sage, and garlic.
Cover with plastic wrap and refrigerate for 3 hours. Heat your grill to the hottest setting.
Grill the turkey drumsticks for about 13 minutes per side. Season with salt and pepper to taste and serve with brown onion. Bon appétit!

Nutrition:
calories: 389
fat: 19.6g
protein: 42.0g
carbs: 6.0g
net carbs: 4.6g
fiber: 1.4g

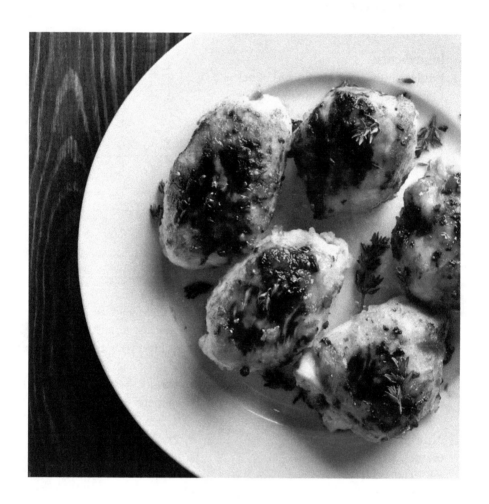

Chicken Meatloaf Cups with Pancetta

Preparation Time: 15 minutes
Cooking Time: 30 minutes
Servings: 6

Ingredients:
2 tbsp. onion, chopped
tsp. garlic, minced
1-pound ground chicken
ounces cooked pancetta, chopped
1 egg, beaten
1 tsp. mustard
Salt and black pepper, to taste
1/2 tsp. crushed red pepper flakes
1 tsp. dried basil
1/2 tsp. dried oregano 4 ounces cheddar cheese, cubed

Directions:
In a mixing bowl, mix mustard, onion, ground turkey, egg, bacon, and garlic. Season with oregano, red pepper, black pepper, basil, and salt. Split the mixture into muffin cups—lower one cube of cheddar cheese into each meatloaf cup. Close the top to cover the cheese. Bake in the oven at 345°F for 20 minutes, or until the meatloaf cups become golden brown.

Nutrition:
Calories: 231
Fat: 10.4g
Fiber: 5.1g
Carbohydrates:3.9 g
Protein: 11.4g

Cheddar Bacon Stuffed Chicken Fillets

Preparation time: 10 minutes
Cooking time: 25 minutes
Servings: 2

Ingredients:
2 chicken fillets, skinless and boneless
½ teaspoon oregano
½ teaspoon tarragon
½ teaspoon paprika
¼ teaspoon ground black pepper
Sea salt, to taste
2 (1-ounce / 28-g) slices bacon
2 (1-ounce / 28-g) slices Cheddar cheese
1 tomato, sliced

Directions:
Sprinkle the chicken fillets with oregano, tarragon, paprika, black pepper, and salt.
Place the bacon slices and cheese on each chicken fillet. Roll up the fillets and secure with toothpicks. Place the stuffed chicken fillets on a lightly greased baking pan. Scatter the sliced tomato around the fillets.
Bake in the preheated oven at 390°F (199°C) for 15 minutes; turn on the other side and bake an additional 5 to 10 minutes or until the meat is no longer pink. Discard the toothpicks and serve immediately. Bon appétit!

Nutrition:
calories: 400
fat: 23.8g
protein: 41.3g
carbs: 3.6g
net carbs: 2.4g
fiber: 1.2g

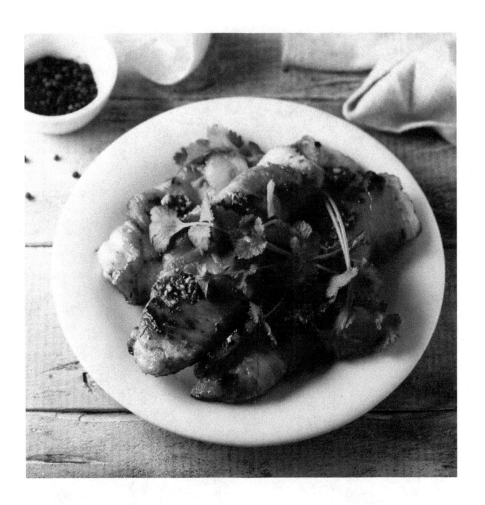

Pork

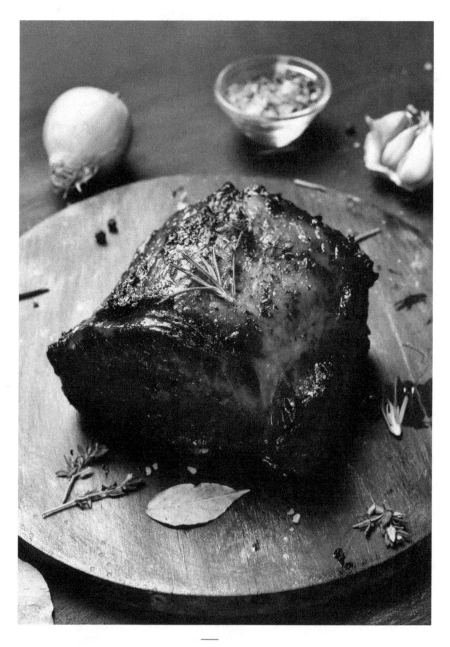

Egg Roll Bowls

Preparation Time: 10minutes
Cooking Time: 30 minutes
Servings: 4

Ingredients:
1 tbsp. vegetable oil
1 clove garlic, minced
1 tbsp. minced fresh ginger
1 lb. ground pork
1 tbsp. sesame oil
1/2 onion, thinly sliced
1 c. shredded carrot
1/4 green cabbage, thinly sliced
1/4 c. soy sauce
1 tbsp. Sriracha
1 green onion, thinly sliced
1 tbsp. sesame seeds

Directions:
Heat oil. Put garlic and ginger and cook until fragrant, about 1 to 2 minutes. Put pork and cook until no pink remains. Push pork to the side and add sesame oil. Put onion, carrot, and cabbage. Stir to combine with meat. Then put soy sauce and Sriracha. Stir and cook until cabbage is tender, about 6 to 8 minutes. Move and mixture to a serving dish Garnish with sesame seeds and the green onions.

Nutrition:
Calories: 321
Fat: 15g
Fiber: 9.5g
Carbohydrates:5.1 g
Protein: 7.4g

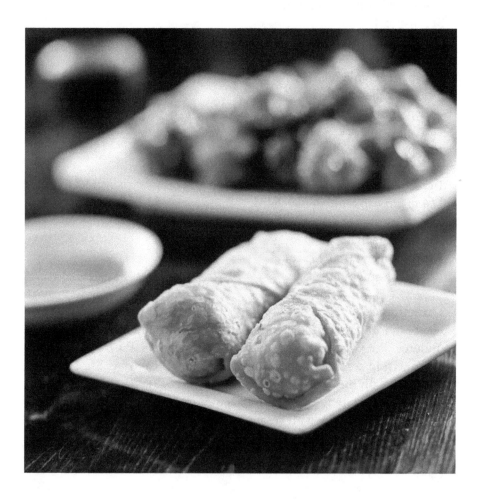

Pickle and Ham Stuffed Pork

Preparation time: 20 minutes
Cooking time: 35 minutes
Servings: 4

Ingredients:
Zest and juice from 2 limes
2 garlic cloves, minced
¾ cup olive oil
1 cup fresh cilantro, chopped
1 cup fresh mint, chopped
teaspoon dried oregano
Salt and black pepper, to taste
teaspoons cumin
4 pork loin steaks
2 pickles, chopped
4 ham slices
6 Swiss cheese slices 2 tablespoons mustard
Salad:
head red cabbage, shredded
tablespoons vinegar
tablespoons olive oil
Salt to taste

Directions:
In a food processor, blitz the lime zest, oil, oregano, black pepper, cumin, cilantro, lime juice, garlic, mint, and salt. Rub the steaks with the mixture and toss well to coat; set aside for some hours in the fridge. Arrange the steaks on a working surface, split the pickles, mustard, cheese, and ham on them, roll, and secure with toothpicks. Heat a pan over medium heat, add in the pork rolls, cook each side for 2 minutes and remove to a baking sheet. Bake in the oven at 350°F (180°C) for 25 minutes. Prepare the red cabbage salad by mixing all salad ingredients and serve with the meat.

Nutrition:
calories: 412 | fat: 37.1g | protein: 25.8g | carbs: 8.1g | net carbs: 3.1g | fiber: 5.0g

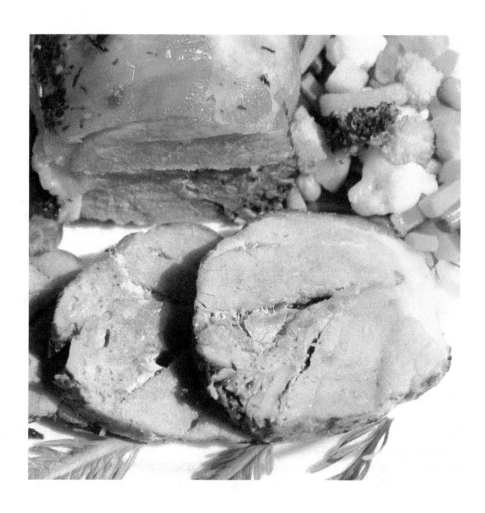

Cheesy Bacon Squash Spaghetti

Preparation Time: 30 minutes
Cooking Time: 50 minutes
Servings: 4

Ingredients:
2 pounds spaghetti squash
2 pounds bacon
1/2 cup of butter
2 cups of shredded parmesan cheese
Salt Black pepper

Directions:
Let the oven preheat to 375F.
Trim or remove each stem of spaghetti squash, slice into rings no more than an inch wide, and take out the seeds. Lay the sliced rings down on the baking sheet, bake for 40-45 minutes. It is ready when the strands separate easily when a fork is used to scrape it. Let it cool. Cook sliced up bacon until crispy. Take out and let it cool. Take off the shell on each ring, separate each strand with a fork, and put them in a bowl. Heat the strands in a microwave to get them warm, then put in butter and stir around till the butter melts. Pour in parmesan cheese and bacon crumbles, and add salt and pepper to your taste. Enjoy.

Nutrition:
Calories: 398
Fat: 12.5g
Fiber: 9.4g
Carbohydrates:4.1 g
Protein: 5.1g

Spiralized Zucchini, Bacon, and Spinach Gratin

Preparation time: 15 minutes
Cooking time: 30 minutes
Servings: 4

Ingredients:
2 large zucchinis, spiralized
4 slices bacon, chopped
2 cups baby spinach
4 ounces (113 g) halloumi cheese, cut into cubes
2 cloves garlic, minced
1 cup heavy cream
½ cup sugar-free tomato sauce
1 cup grated Mozzarella cheese
½ teaspoon dried Italian mixed herbs
Salt and black pepper to taste

Directions:
Preheat the oven to 350°F (180°C). Place the cast iron pan over medium heat and fry the bacon for 4 minutes, then add garlic and cook for 1 minute.
In a bowl, mix the heavy cream, tomato sauce, and ⅙ cup water and add it to the pan. Stir in the zucchini, spinach, halloumi, Italian herbs, salt, and pepper. Sprinkle the Mozzarella cheese on top, and transfer the pan to the oven. Bake for 20 minutes or until the cheese is golden. Serve the gratin warm.

Nutrition:
calories: 351
fat: 27.2g
protein: 15.9g
carbs: 6.6g
net carbs: 5.2g
fiber: 1.4g

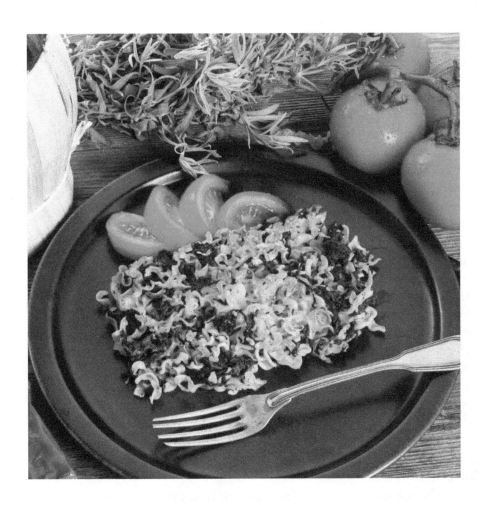

Olla Podrida

Preparation time: 15 minutes
Cooking time: 40 minutes
Servings: 4

Ingredients:
2 tablespoons olive oil
1½ pounds (680 g) pork ribs
yellow onion, chopped
garlic cloves, minced
2 Spanish peppers, chopped
1 Spanish Naga pepper, chopped
1 celery stalk, chopped
½ cup Marsala wine
8 ounces (227 g) button mushrooms, sliced
Sea salt and ground black pepper, to taste
1 teaspoon cayenne pepper
1 cup tomato purée
1 bay laurel

Directions:
Heat 1 tablespoon of the olive oil in a stockpot over medium-high heat. Now, cook the pork ribs for 4 to 5 minutes per side or until brown; set aside.

Then, heat the remaining tablespoon of olive oil and sauté the onion, garlic, peppers, and celery for 5 minutes more or until tender and fragrant.

After that, add in a splash of red wine to scrape up the browned bits that stick to the bottom of the pot.

Add the mushrooms, salt, black pepper, cayenne pepper, tomatoes, and bay laurel to the stockpot.

When the mixture reaches boiling, turn the heat to a medium-low. Add the reserved pork back to the pot. Let it cook, partially covered, for 35 minutes. Serve warm and enjoy!

Nutrition:
calories: 360 | fat: 19.1g | protein: 38.2g | carbs: 4.9g | net carbs: 3.2g | fiber: 1.7g

Bolognese Pork Zoodles

Preparation time: 10 minutes
Cooking time: 25 minutes
Servings: 3

Ingredients:
3 teaspoons olive oil
¾ pound (340 g) ground pork
2 cloves garlic, pressed
2 medium-sized tomatoes, puréed
2 zucchini, spiralized
Heat the olive oil in a saucepan over medium-high heat. Once hot, sear the pork for 3 to 4 minutes or until no longer pink.
Stir in the garlic and cook for 30 seconds more or until fragrant.
Fold in the puréed tomatoes and bring to a boil; immediately turn the heat to medium-low and continue simmering an additional 20 minutes.
After that, fold in the zoodles and continue to cook for a further 1½ minutes until just al dente. Serve hot. Bon appétit!

Nutrition:
calories: 358
fat: 28.6g
protein: 20.2g
carbs: 4.0g
net carbs: 2.8g
fiber: 1.2g

Beef and Lamb

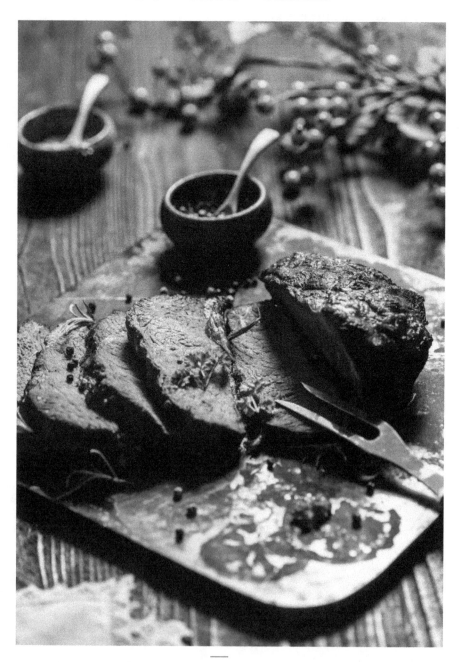

Double Cheese Stuffed Venison

Preparation time: 10 minutes
Cooking time: 25 minutes
Servings: 8

Ingreedients:
2 pounds (907 g) venison tenderloin
2 garlic cloves, minced
2 tablespoons chopped almonds
½ cup Gorgonzola cheese
½ cup Feta cheese
1 teaspoon chopped onion
½ teaspoon salt

Directions:
Preheat your grill to medium. Slice the tenderloin lengthwise to make a pocket for the filling.Combine the rest of the ingredients in a bowl. Stuff the tenderloin with the filling.
Shut the meat with skewers and grill for as long as it takes to reach your desired density.

Nutrition:
calories: 196
fat: 11.9g
protein: 25.1g
carbs: 2.1g
net carbs: 1.6g
fiber: 0.5g

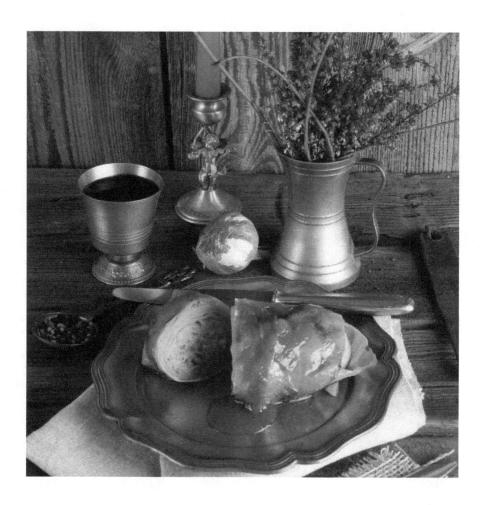

Beef and Veggie Stuffed Butternut Squash

Preparation time: 15 minutes
Cooking time: 60 minutes
Servings: 4

Ingredients:
pounds (907 g) butternut squash, pricked with a fork
Salt and black pepper, to taste
garlic cloves, minced
1 onion, chopped
1 button mushroom, sliced
28 ounces (794 g) canned diced tomatoes
1 teaspoon dried oregano
¼ teaspoon cayenne pepper
½ teaspoon dried thyme
1 pound (454 g) ground beef
1 green bell pepper, chopped

Directions:
Lay the butternut squash on a lined baking sheet, set in the oven at
400°F (205°C), and bake for 40 minutes. After, cut in half, set aside to
let cool, deseed, scoop out most of the flesh and let sit. Heat a greased
pan over medium heat, add in the garlic, mushrooms, onion, and beef,
and cook until the meat browns.
Stir in the green pepper, salt, thyme, tomatoes, oregano, black pepper,
and cayenne, and cook for 10 minutes; stir in the flesh. Stuff the squash
halves with the beef mixture, and bake in the oven for 10 minutes. Split
into plates and enjoy.

Nutrition:
calories: 405
fat: 14.5g
protein: 33.8g
carbs: 20.7g
net carbs: 12.3g
fiber: 8.4g

Hungarian Beef and Carrot Goulash

Preparation time: 15 minutes
Cooking time: 9 to 10 hours
Servings: 6

Ingredients:
1 tablespoon extra-virgin olive oil
1½ pounds (680 g) beef, cut into 1-inch pieces
½ sweet onion, chopped
1 carrot, cut into ½-inch-thick slices
red bell pepper, diced
teaspoons minced garlic
1 cup beef broth
¼ cup tomato paste
1 tablespoon Hungarian paprika
1 bay leaf
cup sour cream
tablespoons chopped fresh parsley, for garnish

Directions:
Lightly grease the insert of the slow cooker with the olive oil.
Add the beef, onion, carrot, red bell pepper, garlic, broth, tomato paste,
paprika, and bay leaf to the insert.
Cover and cook on low for 9 to 10 hours.
Remove the bay leaf and stir in the sour cream.
Serve topped with the parsley.

Nutrition:
calories: 550
fat: 41.9g
protein: 31.8g
carbs: 7.9g
net carbs: 5.8g
fiber: 2.1g

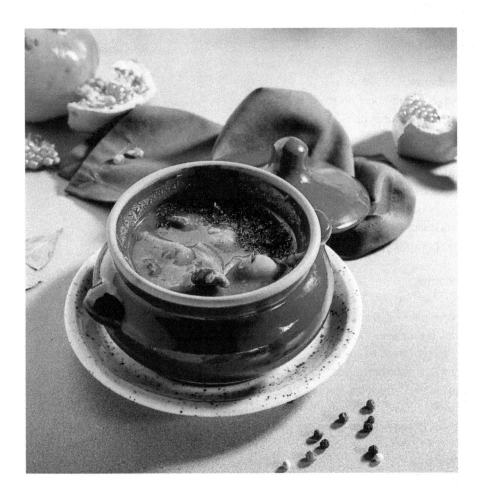

Lemony Beef Rib Roast

Preparation time: 15 minutes
Cooking time: 35 minutes
Servings: 6

Ingredients:
5 pounds (2.3 kg) beef rib roast, on the bone
3 heads garlic, cut in half
3 tablespoons olive oil
6 shallots, peeled and halved
lemons, zested and juiced
tablespoons mustard seeds
3 tablespoons Swerve
Salt and black pepper to taste
3 tablespoons thyme leaves

Directions:
Preheat oven to 450°F (235°C). Place garlic heads and shallots in a roasting dish, toss with olive oil, and bake for 15 minutes. Pour lemon juice on them. Score shallow crisscrosses patterns on the meat and set aside.

Mix Swerve, mustard seeds, thyme, salt, pepper, and lemon zest to make a rub; and apply it all over the beef. Place the beef on the shallots and garlic; cook in the oven for 15 minutes. Reduce the heat to 400°F (205°C), cover the dish with foil, and continue cooking for 5 minutes.

Once ready, remove the dish, and let sit covered for 15 minutes before slicing.

Per Serving
calories: 555
fat: 38.5g
protein: 58.3g
carbs: 7.7g
net carbs: 2.4g
fiber: 5.3g

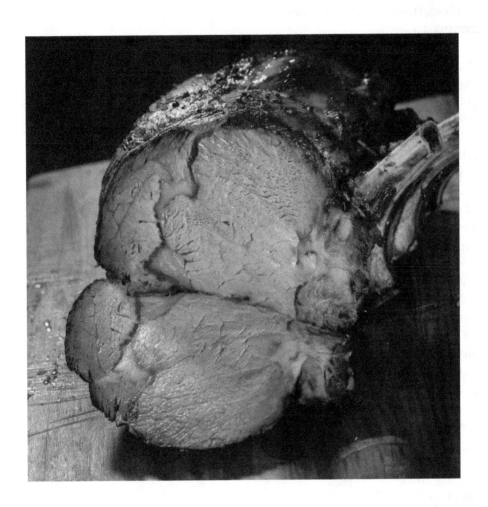

Veal, Mushroom, and Green Bean Stew

Preparation time: 15 minutes
Cooking time: 1 hour 55 minutes
Servings: 6

Ingredients:
tablespoons olive oil
pounds (1.4 kg) veal shoulder, cubed
1 onion, chopped
1 garlic clove, minced
Salt and black pepper, to taste
1 cup water
1½ cups red wine
12 ounces (340 g) canned tomato sauce
1 carrot, chopped
cup mushrooms, chopped
½ cup green beans
teaspoons dried oregano

Directions:
Set a pot over medium heat and warm the oil. Brown the veal for 5-6 minutes. Stir in the onion, and garlic, and cook for 3 minutes. Place in the wine, oregano, carrot, black pepper, salt, tomato sauce, water, and mushrooms, bring to a boil, reduce the heat to low. Cook for 1 hour and 45 minutes, then add in the green beans and cook for 5 minutes. Adjust the seasoning and split among serving bowls to serve.

Nutrition:
calories: 416
fat: 21.1g
protein: 44.2g
carbs: 7.3g
net carbs: 5.1g
fiber: 2.2g

Hot Beef Curry with Bok Choy

Preparation time: 10 minutes
Cooking time: 7 to 8 hours
Servings: 6

Ingredients:
1 tablespoon extra-virgin olive oil
1 pound (454 g) beef chuck roast, cut into 2-inch pieces
1 sweet onion, chopped
red bell pepper, diced
cups coconut milk
2 tablespoons hot curry powder
tablespoon coconut aminos
teaspoons grated fresh ginger
2 teaspoons minced garlic
1 cup shredded baby bok choy

Directions:
Lightly grease the insert of the slow cooker with the olive oil.
Add the beef, onion, and bell pepper to the insert.
In a medium bowl, whisk together the coconut milk, curry, coconut aminos, ginger, and garlic. Pour the sauce into the insert and stir to combine.
Cover and cook on low for 7 to 8 hours.
Stir in the bok choy and let stand 15 minutes.
Serve warm.

Nutrition:
calories: 505
fat: 41.8g
protein: 22.9g
carbs: 9.8g
net carbs: 6.8g
fiber: 3.0g

Fish and Seafood

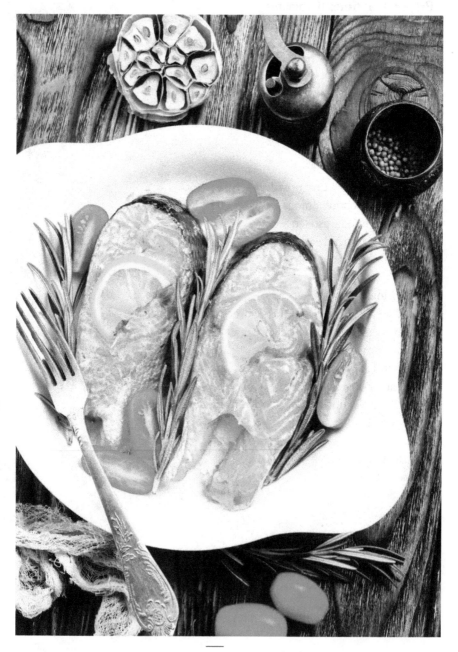

Sage Shrimps

Preparation time: 10 minutes
Cooking time: 1 hours
Servings: 4

Ingredients:
1-pound shrimps, peeled
1 teaspoon dried sage
1 teaspoon minced garlic
1 teaspoon white pepper 1 cup tomatoes chopped
½ cup of water

Directions
Put all ingredients in the slow cooker and close the lid.
Cook the shrimps on High for 1 hour.

Nutrition
146 calories,
26.4g protein,
4.1g carbohydrates,
2.1g fat,
0.8g fiber,
239mg cholesterol,
280mg sodium,
310mg potassium.

Butter Salmon

Preparation time: 10 minutes
Cooking time: 1.5 hours
Servings: 2

Ingredients:
8 oz. salmon fillet
3 tablespoons butter
1 teaspoon dried sage
¼ cup of water

Directions
Churn butter with sage and preheat the mixture until liquid.
Then cut the salmon fillets into 2 servings and put in the slow cooker.
Add water and melted butter mixture.
Close the lid and cook the salmon on High for 1.5 hours.

Nutrition
304 calories,
22.2g protein,
0.2g carbohydrates,
24.3g fat,
0.1g fiber
, 96mg cholesterol,
174mg sodium,
444mg potassium.

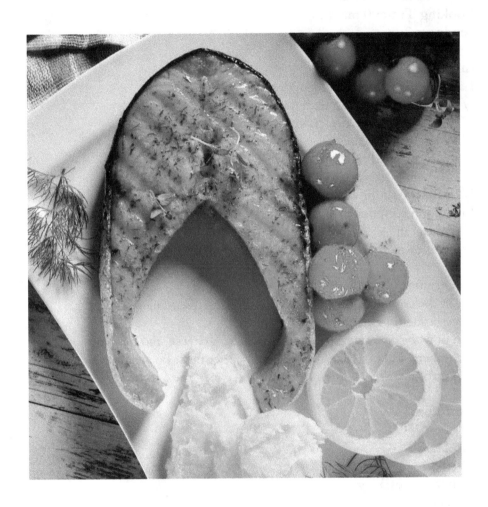

Crab-stuffed Avocado

Preparation Time: 20 minutes
Cooking Time: 0 minutes
Servings: 2

Ingredients:
1 avocado, peeled, halved lengthwise, and pitted
1/2 teaspoon freshly squeezed lemon juice
41/2 ounces Dungeness crabmeat
1/2 cup cream cheese
1/4 cup chopped red bell pepper
1/4 cup chopped, peeled English cucumber
1/2 scallion, chopped
1 teaspoon chopped cilantro
Pinch sea salt
Freshly ground black pepper

Directions:
Brush the cut edges of the avocado with the lemon juice and set the halves aside on a plate.
In a bowl or container, the crabmeat, cream cheese, red pepper, cucumber, scallion, cilantro, salt, and pepper must be well mixed.
The crab mixture will then be divided between the avocado

Nutrition:
Calories: 239
Fat: 11.4g
Fiber: 8.1g
Carbohydrates:3.8 g
Protein: 5.9g

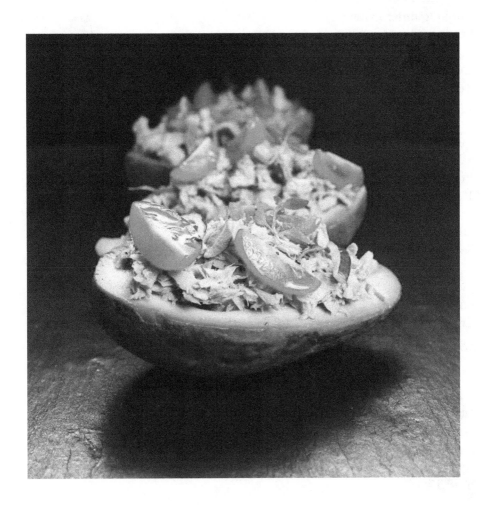

Tilapia and Red Cabbage Taco Bowl

Preparation time: 10 minutes
Cooking time: 15 minutes
Servings: 4

Ingredients:
2 cups cauli rice
2 teaspoons butter
4 tilapia fillets, cut into cubes
¼ teaspoon taco seasoning
Salt and chili pepper to taste
¼ head red cabbage, shredded
1 ripe avocado, pitted and chopped

Directions:
Sprinkle cauli rice in a bowl with a little water and microwave for 3 minutes. Fluff after with a fork and set aside. Melt butter in a skillet over medium heat, rub the tilapia with the taco seasoning, salt, and chili pepper, and fry until brown on all sides, for about 8 minutes in total.
Transfer to a plate and set aside. In 4 serving bowls, share the cauli rice, cabbage, fish, and avocado. Serve with chipotle lime sour cream dressing.

Nutrition:
calories: 270
fat: 23.5g
protein: 16.6g
carbs: 9.1g
net carbs: 3.9g
fiber: 5.2g

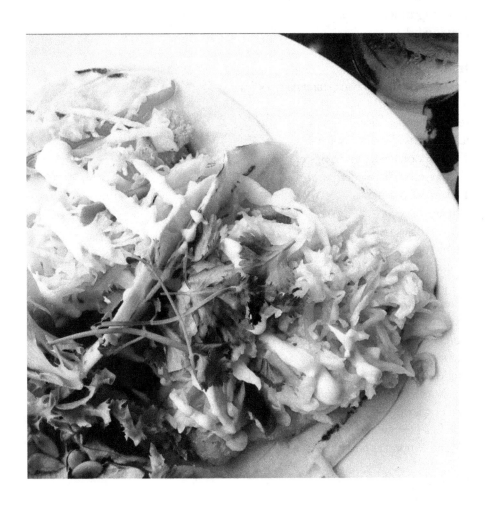

Tuna Shirataki Pad Thai

Preparation time: 15 minutes
Cooking time: 5 minutes
Servings: 4

Ingredients:
1 (7-ounce / 198-g) pack shirataki noodles
4 cups water
red bell pepper, sliced
tablespoons soy sauce, sugar-free
1 tablespoon ginger-garlic paste
1 teaspoon chili powder
1 tablespoon water
4 tuna steaks
Salt and black pepper to taste
1 tablespoon olive oil
1 tablespoon parsley, chopped

Directions:
In a colander, rinse the shirataki noodles with running cold water.
Bring a pot of salted water to a boil; blanch the noodles for 2 minutes. Drain and set aside.
Preheat a grill on medium-high. Season the tuna with salt and black pepper, brush with olive oil, and grill covered. Cook for 3 minutes on each side.
In a bowl, whisk soy sauce, ginger-garlic paste, olive oil, chili powder, and water. Add bell pepper, and noodles and toss to coat.
Assemble noodles and tuna in serving plate and garnish with parsley.

Nutrition:
calories: 288
fat: 16.1g
protein: 23.2g
carbs: 7.7g
net carbs: 6.7g
fiber: 1.0g

Crab Patties

Preparation time: 10 minutes
Cooking time: 5 minutes
Servings: 8

Ingredients:
2 tablespoons coconut oil
1 tablespoon lemon juice
cup lump crab meat
teaspoons Dijon mustard
1 egg, beaten
1½ tablespoons coconut flour

Directions:
In a bowl to the crabmeat, add all the ingredients, except for the oil; mix well to combine. Make patties out of the mixture. Melt the coconut oil in a skillet over medium heat. Add the crab patties and cook for about 2-3 minutes per side.

Nutrition:
calories: 216
fat: 11.6g
protein: 15.2g
carbs: 3.6g
net carbs: 3.5g
fiber: 0.1g

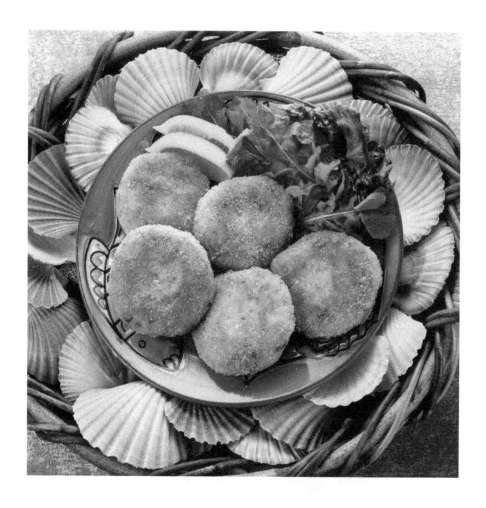

Soups

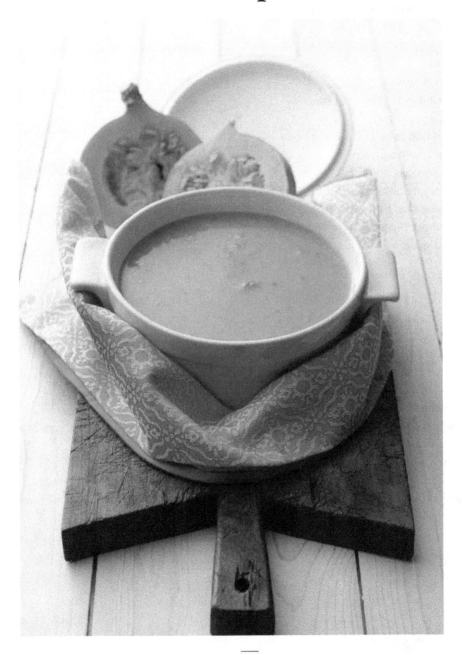

Cauliflower and Lamb Soup

Preparation time: 10 minutes
Cooking time: 4 hours
Servings: 6

Ingredients:
1 pound (454 g) ground lamb
5 cups beef broth
1 cauliflower head, cut into florets
1 cup heavy cream
yellow onion, chopped
cloves garlic, chopped
1 tablespoon freshly chopped thyme
½ teaspoon cracked black pepper
½ teaspoon salt

Directions:
Add the ground lamb and cauliflower to the base of a stockpot.
Add in the remaining ingredients minus the heavy cream, and cook on high for 4 hours.
Warm the heavy cream before adding to the soup. Use an immersion blender to blend the soup until creamy.

Nutrition:
calories: 264
fat: 14.0g
protein: 26.9g
carbs: 5.9g
net carbs: 3.9g
fiber: 2.0g

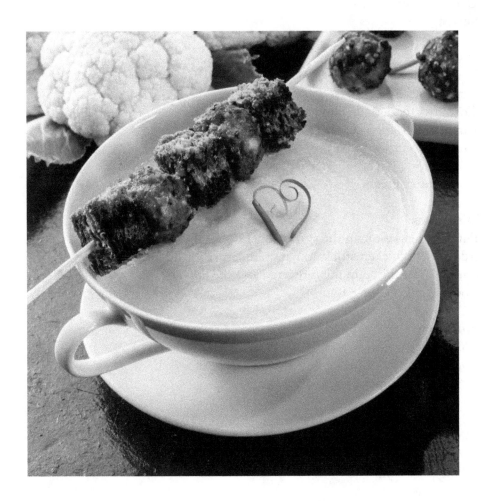

Barley Soup

Preparation time: 10 minutes
Cooking time: 8 hours
Servings: 5

Ingredients:
¼ cup barley
5 cups chicken stock
4 oz. pork tenderloin, chopped
1 tablespoon dried cilantro
1 tablespoon tomato paste
3 oz. carrot, grated
½ cup heavy cream

Directions:
Put pork tenderloin in the slow cooker.
Add barley, chicken stock, tomato paste, carrot, and heavy cream.
Carefully stir the soup mixture and close the lid.
Cook it on Low for 8 hours.

Nutrition:
126 calories,
8.3g protein,
10.1g carbohydrates,
6g fat,
2.2g fiber,
33mg cholesterol,
797mg sodium,
249mg potassium.

Chorizo Soup

Preparation time: 10 minutes
Cooking time: 5 hours
Servings: 6

Ingredients:
9 oz. chorizo, chopped
7 cups of water
1 cup potato, chopped
1 teaspoon minced garlic, chopped
1 zucchini, chopped
½ cup spinach, chopped
1 teaspoon salt

Directions:
Put the chorizo in the skillet and roast it for 2 minutes per side on high heat.
Then transfer the chorizo in the slow cooker.
Add water, potato, minced garlic, zucchini, spinach, and salt.
Close the lid and cook the soup on high for 5 hours.
Then cool the soup to the room temperature.

Nutrition:
210 calories,
11g protein,
4.3g carbohydrates,
16.4g fat,
0.7g fiber,
37mg cholesterol,
927mg sodium,
326mg potassium.

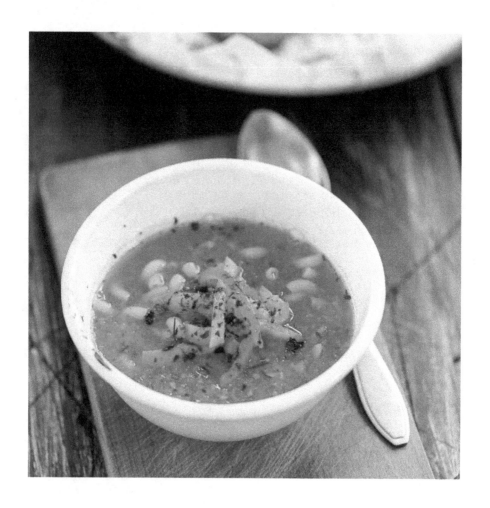

Avocado and Cucumber Soup 20

Preparation time: 10 minutes
Cooking time: 0 minutes
Servings: 4

Ingredients:
1 ripe avocado
½ cucumber, sliced
1 cup full-fat unsweetened coconut milk
1 tablespoon freshly chopped mint leaves
1 tablespoon freshly squeezed lemon juice
Pinch of salt

Directions:
Add all the ingredients to a high-speed blender and blend until creamy.
Chill in the refrigerator for 1 hour before serving.

Nutrition:
calories: 250
fat: 24.1g
protein: 2.9g
carbs: 8.9g
net carbs: 4.1g
fiber: 4.8g

New England Clam Chowder

Preparation Time: 15 minutes
Cooking Time: 25 minutes
Servings: 2

Ingredients:
2 bacon slices, chopped
1 celery stalk, chopped
1/4 medium onion, chopped
1 garlic clove, minced
cup chicken broth
(6.5-ounce) cans chopped clams, drained, juices reserved
1 medium kohlrabi, peeled and cubed
1 bay leaf
1/2 teaspoon pink Himalayan sea salt
1/4 teaspoon freshly ground black pepper
1/4 teaspoon dried thyme
Pinch of ground white pepper
11/2 cups decadent (whipping) cream

Directions:
Cook bacon. The pot with the bacon grease, sauté the celery and onion
for 8 to 10 minutes until the onion is translucent. Add the garlic. Add
the broth, reserved clam juice (not the clams yet), the kohlrabi, bay leaf,
salt, black pepper, thyme, and white pepper. Simmer for 10 to 15
minutes, until the kohlrabi is tender. Add the cream and clams. Stir to
combine. Simmer the soup for roughly 20 minutes, or until it reduces
to your desired consistency. Remove and discard the bay leaf. Stir in
the bacon crumbles and serve.

Nutrition:
Calories: 376
Fat: 15.9g
Fiber: 10g
Carbohydrates:4.1 g
Protein: 13.1g

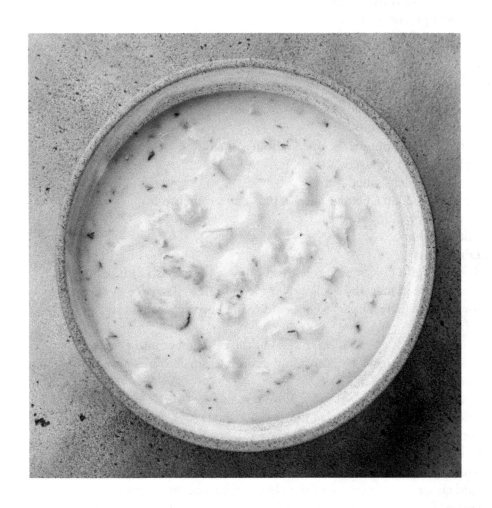

Bacon and Cauliflower Soup

Preparation time: 15 minutes
Cooking time: 4 or 8 hours
Servings: 5

Ingredients:
10 slices bacon
2 large or 3 small heads cauliflower
4 cups chicken broth
½ large yellow onion, chopped (about 1⅓ cups)
3 cloves garlic, pressed
¼ cup (½ stick) salted butter
2 cups shredded Cheddar cheese, plus extra for garnish
1 cup heavy whipping cream
Salt and pepper
Directions:
Snipped fresh chives or sliced green onions, for garnish (optional) 1
Fry the bacon in a large skillet over medium heat. Transfer to a paper
towel–lined plate, allow to cool, and then chop. Set aside in the
refrigerator.
Core the heads of cauliflower and cut the cauliflower into florets. Place
the florets in a food processor and chop into small to mediumsized
pieces. (Don't rice it.)
In a large slow cooker (I use a 5½-quart slow cooker), combine the
chicken broth, onion, garlic, butter, and cauliflower. Stir, cover, and
cook on high for 4 hours or on low for 8 hours. Once the cauliflower
is tender, switch the slow cooker to the keep warm setting and use a
whisk to stir and mash the cauliflower to a smooth consistency.
Add about three-quarters of the chopped bacon, the cheese, and the
cream. Season with salt and pepper to taste. Stir well until the cheese is
melted.
Serve garnished with additional cheese, the remaining bacon, and
chives or green onions, if desired.
Nutrition:
calories: 283 | fat: 22.1g | protein: 11.9g | carbs: 8.1g | net carbs: 6.2g
| fiber: 1.9g

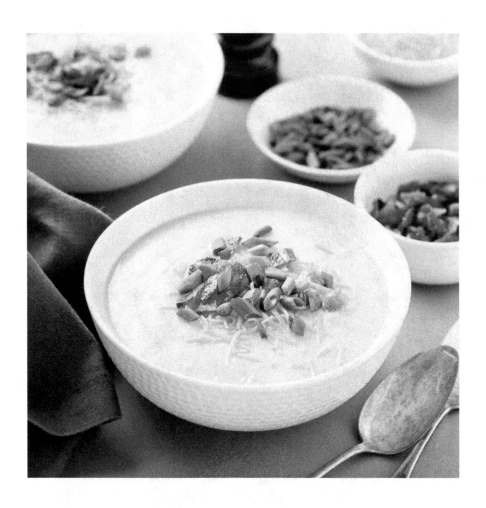

Snacks and Appetizers

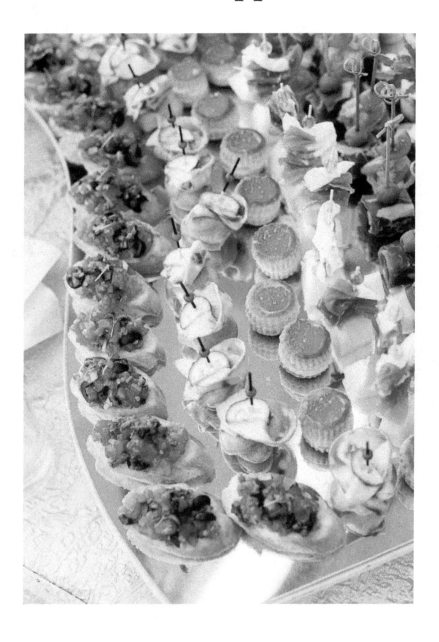

Keto Trail Mix

Preparation Time: 5 minutes
Cooking Time: 0 minutes
Servings: 3

Ingredients:
1/2 cup salted pumpkin seeds
1/2 cup slivered almonds
3/4 cup roasted pecan halves
3/4 cup unsweetened cranberries
1 cup toasted coconut flakes

Directions:
In a skillet, place almonds and pecans. Heat for 2-3 minutes and let cool.
Once cooled, in a large resealable plastic bag, combine all ingredients.
Seal and shake vigorously to mix.
Evenly divide into suggested servings and store in airtight meal prep containers.

Nutrition:
Calories: 98
Fat: 1.2g
Fiber: 4.1g
Carbohydrates:1.1 g
Protein: 3.2g

Spanish Sausage and Cheese Stuffed Mushrooms

Preparation time: 15 minutes
Cooking time: 25 minutes
Servings: 6

Ingredients:
30 button mushrooms, stalks removed and cleaned
8 ounces (227 g) Chorizo sausage, crumbled
2 scallions, chopped
2 green garlic stalks, chopped
2 tablespoons fresh parsley, chopped
10 ounces (283 g) goat cheese, crumbled
Sea salt and ground black pepper, to season
½ teaspoon red pepper flakes, crushed

Directions:
Place the mushroom caps on a lightly greased baking sheet.
Mix the remaining ingredients until well combined. Divide this stuffing between the mushroom caps.
Bake in the preheated oven at 340°F (171°C) for 25 minutes or until thoroughly cooked. Serve with cocktail sticks. Bon appétit!

Nutrition:
calories: 325
fat: 23.6g
protein: 23.0g
carbs: 5.0g
net carbs: 3.8g
fiber: 1.2g

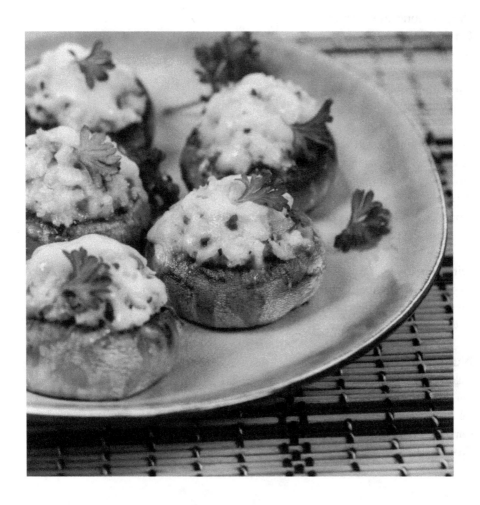

Lemon Shrimp Dip

Preparation time: 10 minutes
Cooking time: 2 hours
Servings: 2

Ingredients:
3 ounces cream cheese, soft
½ cup heavy cream
pound shrimp, peeled, deveined and chopped
½ tablespoon balsamic vinegar
tablespoons mayonnaise½ tablespoon lemon juice
A pinch of salt and black pepper
2 ounces mozzarella, shredded
1 tablespoon parsley, chopped

Directions:
In your slow cooker, mix the cream cheese with the shrimp, heavy cream and the other ingredients, whisk, put the lid on and cook on Low for 2 hours. Divide into bowls and serve as a dip.

Nutrition
Calories 342,
Fat 4,
Fiber 3,
Carbs 7,
Protein 10

Artichokes Spinach Spread

Preparation time: 10 minutes
Cooking time: 2 hours
Servings: 2

Ingredients:
ounces spinach
ounces canned artichokes hearts, drained and chopped
2 tablespoons mayonnaise
2 ounces Alfredo sauce
A pinch of salt and black pepper
1 ounce Swiss cheese, shredded

Directions:
In your slow cooker, mix spinach with artichokes, mayo, Alfredo sauce, salt, pepper and Swiss cheese, stir, cover and cook on Low for 2 hours.
Serve as a party spread.
Enjoy!

Nutrition
Calories 132,
Fat 4,
Fiber 3,
Carbs 10,
Protein 4

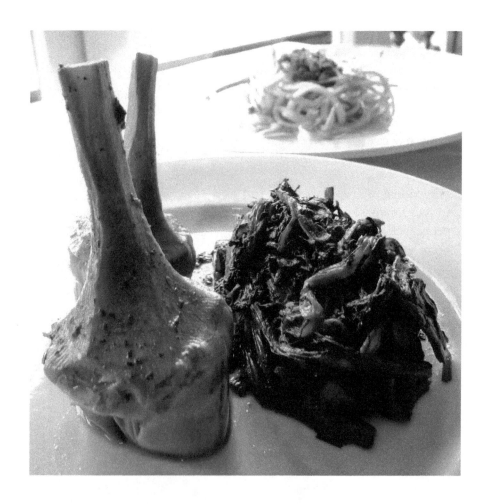

Apple Dip

Preparation time: 10 minutes
Cooking time: 1 hour and 30 minutes
Servings: 8

Ingredients:
5 apples, peeled and chopped
½ teaspoon cinnamon powder
12 ounces jarred caramel sauce
A pinch of nutmeg, ground

Directions:
In your slow cooker, mix apples with cinnamon, caramel sauce and nutmeg, stir, cover and cook on High for 1 hour and 30 minutes.
Divide into bowls and serve.

Nutrition
Calories 200,
Fat 3,
Fiber 6,
Carbs 10, Protein 5

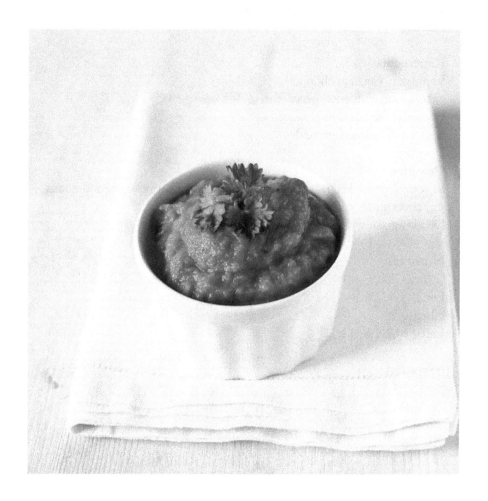

Monterrey Jack Cheese Chips

Preparation time: 10 minutes
Cooking time: 15 minutes
Servings: 4

Ingredients:
2 cups Monterrey Jack cheese, grated
Salt to taste
½ teaspoon garlic powder
½ teaspoon cayenne pepper
½ teaspoon dried rosemary

Directions:
Mix grated cheese with spices. Create 2 tablespoons of cheese mixture into small mounds on a lined baking sheet. Bake for about 15 minutes at 425°F (220°C); then allow to cool to harden the chips.

Nutrition:
calories: 439
fat: 36.9g
protein: 26.9g
carbs: 1.8g
net carbs: 1.7g
fiber: 0.1g

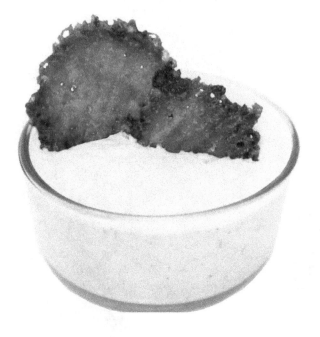

Dessert

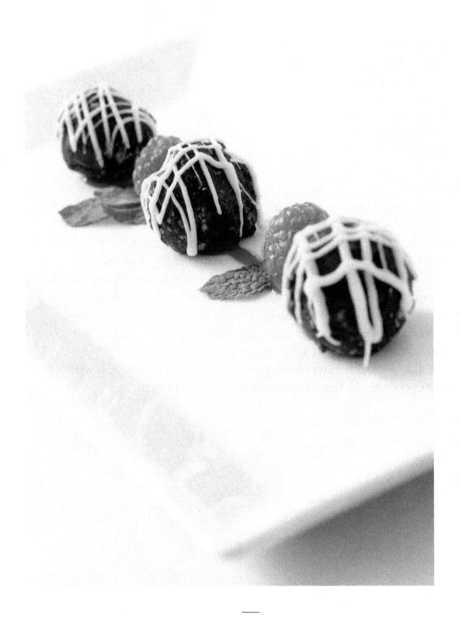

PB& J Cups

Preparation Time: 20 minutes
Cooking Time: 5 minutes
Servings: 4

Ingredients:
1/4 cup of water
1 teaspoon gelatin
3/4 cup of coconut oil
3/4 cup raspberries
6 to 8 tablespoon Stevia
3/4 cup peanut butter

Directions:
Line a muffin pan with parchment paper. In a pan, combine the raspberries and water over medium heat. Bring to a boil and then reduce the heat and let the water dry. Mash the berries with a fork. Add in 2 to 4 tablespoons of the powdered sweetener. Add in the gelatin and set aside to cool. Now make peanut butter mixture. In the pan, put the peanut butter and coconut oil. Cook for 30 to 60 seconds, until melted. Also, add in 2 to 4 tablespoons of the powdered sweetener. Put half of the peanut butter mixture in a muffin pan and put in the freezer to firm up about 15 minutes.
Divide the raspberry mixture among the muffin cups and top with the remaining peanut butter mixture. Refrigerate until firm.

Nutrition:
Calories: 191
Fat: 6.1g
Fiber: 2.2g
Carbohydrates:1.8 g
Protein: 3.1g

Bread and Berries Pudding

Preparation time: 10 minutes
Cooking time: 3 hours
Servings: 2

Ingredients:
2 cups white bread, cubed
cup blackberries
tablespoons butter, melted
2 tablespoons white sugar
cup almond milk
¼ cup heavy cream
eggs, whisked
1 tablespoon lemon zest, grated
¼ teaspoon vanilla extract

Directions:
In your slow cooker, mix the bread with the berries, butter and the other ingredients, toss gently, put the lid on and cook on Low for 3 hours. Divide pudding between dessert plates and serve.

Nutrition:
Calories 354,
Fat 12,
Fiber 4,
Carbs 29,
Protein 11

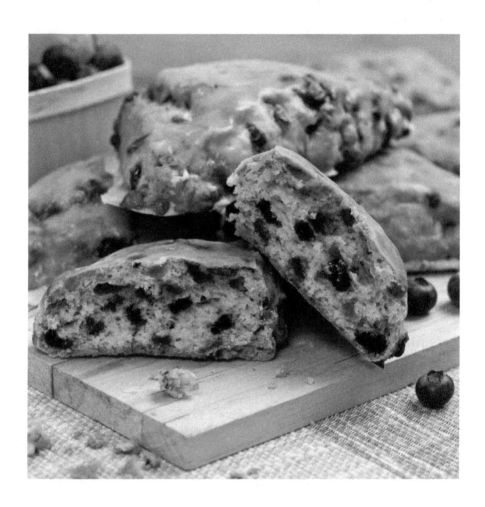

Orange Marmalade

Preparation time: 10 minutes
Cooking time: 3 hours
Servings: 8

Ingredients:
Juice of 2 lemons
3 pounds sugar
1 pound oranges, peeled and cut into segments
1-pint water

Directions:
In your slow cooker, mix lemon juice with sugar, oranges and water, cover and cook on High for 3 hours.
Stir one more time, divide into cups and serve cold.

Nutrition
Calories 100,
Fat 4,
Fiber 4,
Carbs 12,
Protein 4

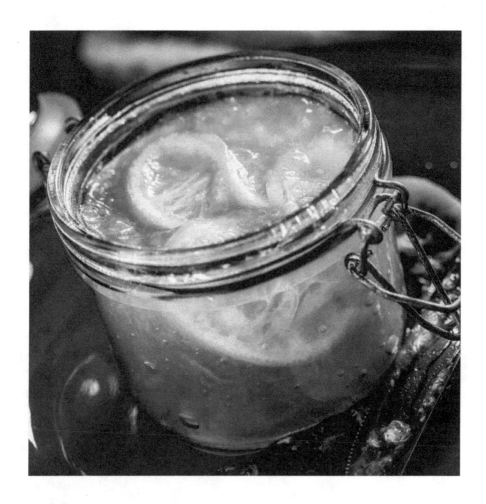

Penuche Bars

Preparation time: 15 minutes
Cooking: time: 0 minutes
Servings: 10

Ingredients:
½ stick butter
2 tablespoons tahini (sesame paste)
½ cup almond butter
teaspoon Stevia
ounces (57 g) baker's chocolate, sugar-free
A pinch of salt
A pinch of grated nutmeg
½ teaspoon cinnamon powder

Directions:
Microwave the butter for 30 to 35 seconds. Fold in the tahini, almond butter, Stevia, and chocolate.
Sprinkle with salt, nutmeg, and cinnamon; whisk to combine well. Scrape the mixture into a parchment-lined baking tray.
Transfer to the freezer for 40 minutes. Cut into bars and enjoy!

Nutrition:
calories: 180
fat: 18.4g
protein: 1.7g
carbs: 3.1g
net carbs: 2.0g
fiber: 1.1g

Meringues

Preparation time: 20 minutes
Cooking time: 2 hours
Makes: 30

Ingredients:
4 large egg whites
¼ teaspoon cream of tartar
¼ teaspoon sea salt
½ cup granulated erythritol-monk fruit blend
¼ cup powdered erythritol-monk fruit blend
½ teaspoon vanilla extract

Directions:
Preheat the oven to 200°F (93°C). Line the baking sheet with parchment paper and set aside.

In the large bowl, using an electric mixer on medium, beat the egg whites, cream of tartar, and salt for 1 to 2 minutes, until foamy and the egg whites just begin to turn opaque.

Continue to whip the egg whites, adding in the granulated and powdered erythritol–monk fruit blend about 1 teaspoon at a time and scraping the bowl once or twice.

Once all the erythritol–monk fruit blend has been added, increase the mixer speed to high and whip for 5 to 7 minutes, until the meringue is glossy and very stiff. Using a rubber spatula, gently fold in the vanilla.

Scoop the meringue into the pastry bag fitted with a French star tip and pipe 2-inch-diameter kisses onto the prepared baking sheet.

Alternatively, spoon the meringue onto the sheet for a more organic shape.

Bake for 2 hours, or until crisp and lightly browned. Allow to cool completely on the cooling rack before serving. Leftovers can be stored in an airtight, nonporous container at room temperature for about 1 week.

Nutrition: (3 Meringues)
calories: 8 | fat: 0g | protein: 2.0g | carbs: 0g | net carbs: 0g | fiber: 0g

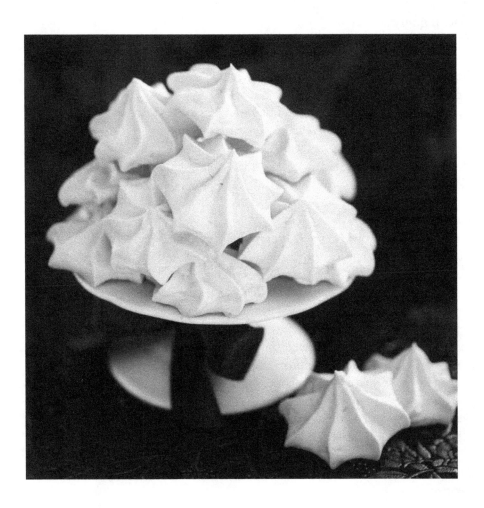

Strawberry Mousse

Preparation time: 10 minutes
Cooking time: 0 minutes
Servings: 6

Ingredients:
8 ounces (227 g) strawberries, sliced
¼ cup granulated erythritol–monk fruit blend; less sweet: 2 tablespoons
½ ounce (14 g) full-fat cream cheese, at room temperature
1 cup heavy whipping cream, divided
⅛ teaspoon vanilla extract
⅛ teaspoon salt

Directions:
Put the large metal bowl in the freezer to chill for at least 5 minutes.
In a blender or food processor, purée the strawberries and erythritol– monk fruit blend. Set aside.
In the chilled large bowl, using an electric mixer on medium high,
beat the cream cheese and ¼ cup of heavy cream until well combined, stopping and scraping the bowl once or twice, as needed. Add the vanilla and salt and mix to combine. Add the remaining ¾ cup of heavy cream and beat on high for 1 to 3 minutes, until very stiff peaks form.
Gently fold the purée into the whipped cream. Refrigerate for at least 1 hour and up to overnight before serving.
Serve in short glasses or small mason jars.
Store leftovers in an airtight container for up to 5 days in the refrigerator.

Nutrition:
calories: 160
fat: 15.9g
protein: 0.9g
carbs: 4.0g
net carbs: 3.0g
fiber: 1.0g

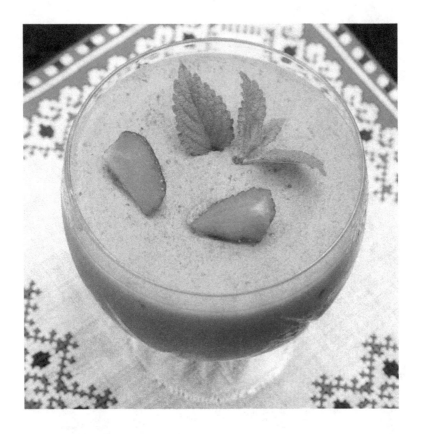

Drinks

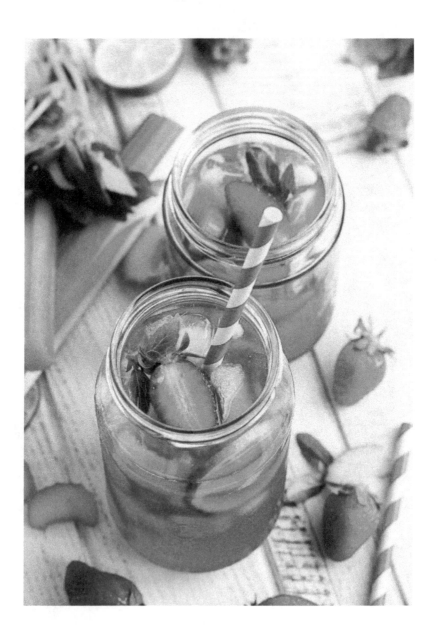

Banana Smoothie

Preparation Time: 10 minutes
Cooking Time: 0 minutes
Servings: 2

Ingredients:
11/2 cups unsweetened almond milk
1/2 cup heavy (whipping) cream
banana
scoops (25–28 grams) vanilla protein powder
2 tablespoons tahini
1/2 teaspoon ground cinnamon
5 ice cubes

Directions:
Blend the smoothie. Put the almond milk, cream, banana, protein powder, tahini, cinnamon, and ice in a blender and blend until smooth and creamy. Serve. Pour into two tall glasses and serve.

Nutrition:
Calories: 308
Fat: 4.2g
Fiber: 9.5g
Carbohydrates:2.2 g
Protein: 7.4g

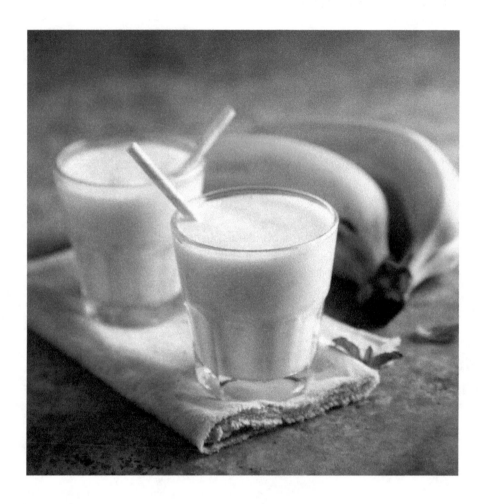

Scallion Ginger Dressing

Preparation time: 8 minutes
Cooking time: 0 minutes
Makes: ¾ cup

Ingredients:
¼ cup chopped scallions
3 tablespoons avocado oil or other light-tasting oil
2 tablespoons filtered water
2 tablespoons fish sauce (no sugar added)
2 tablespoons granulated erythritol
1 tablespoon lime juice
1 tablespoon white vinegar
1 tablespoon peeled and minced fresh ginger
1 teaspoon toasted sesame oil

Direction:
Place all of the ingredients in a small blender and blend until mostly smooth. Store in an airtight container in the refrigerator for up to 1 week.

Nutrition:
calories: 76
fat: 8.0g
protein: 1.0g
carbs: 1.0g
net carbs: 1.0g
fiber: 0g

Cajun Seasoning

Preparation time: 5 minutes
Cooking time: 0 minutes
Makes: ⅓ cup

Ingredients:
1 tablespoon garlic powder
1 tablespoon kosher salt
tablespoon paprika
teaspoons cayenne pepper
2 teaspoons dried oregano leaves
2 teaspoons dried thyme leaves
2 teaspoons onion powder
1 teaspoon ground black pepper

Directions:
Place all of the ingredients in a small bowl and mix well. Store in an airtight container for up to 6 months.

Nutrition:
calories: 5
fat: 0g
protein: 0g
carbs: 1.0g
net carbs: 1.0g
fiber: 0g

Pumpkin Spice Latte

Preparation Time: 5-10 minutes
Cooking Time: 0 minutes
Servings: 1

Ingredients:
ounce of unsalted butter
tablespoons of pumpkin spice
2 tablespoons of instant coffee powder
1 cup of boiling water
Heavy whipped cream

Directions:
Put all ingredients except cream inside a blender, and blend until the foam is formed.
Pour in a cup, and sprinkle cinnamon.
Add a dollop of cream and enjoy hot.

Nutrition:
Calories: 217
Fat: 12.9
Fiber: 2.3g
Carbohydrates:3.1 g
Protein:4.1 g

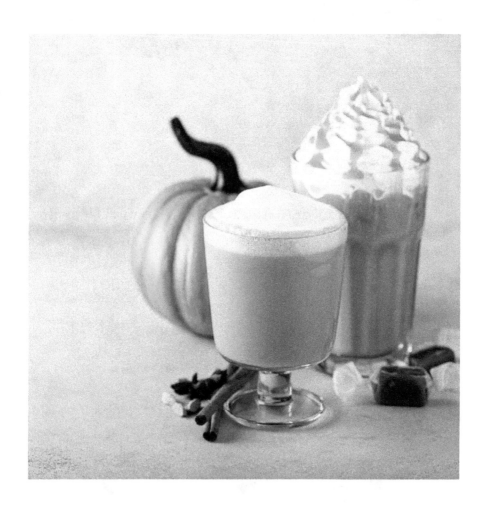

Beef Seasoning

Preparation time: 5 minutes
Cooking time: 0 minutes
Makes: ½ cup

Ingredients:
2 tablespoons kosher salt
1 tablespoon garlic powder
1 tablespoon ground black pepper
1 tablespoon onion powder
1 tablespoon smoked paprika
1 teaspoon dried thyme leaves
1 teaspoon ground coriander
1 teaspoon ground cumin

Direction:
Place all of the ingredients in a small bowl and mix well. Store in an airtight container for up to 6 months.

Nutrition:
calories: 4 fat: 0g
protein: 0g
carbs: 1.5g
net carbs: 1.0g
fiber: 0.5g

CPSIA information can be obtained
at www.ICGtesting.com
Printed in the USA
BVHW061036220321
603178BV00004B/234

9 781914 450242